My Natural Weight-loss Recipe

Learn the Basic Ingredients to Losing Weight Naturally for Life.

By Irina Dura

Published in 2020

Edition 2

Website: www.myweightlossjourneytips.com

From the Author of:

<u>My 18 Year Weight-loss Journey – How I Finally Lost 35kg (77 pounds) While Still Enjoying My Favorite Food</u>

Get your copy of 'My 18 Year Weight-loss Journey' on Amazon:

www.amazon.com/author/irinadura

ISBN: 978-0-6480520-7-4

Copyright

Copyright © 2020 Irina Dura.

All Rights Reserved. My Natural Weight-loss Recipe

No part of this publication may be used or reproduced for any means, graphic, electronic or mechanical, including photocopying, recording, taping or by any information storage retrieval system without the written permission of the author.

Because of the dynamic nature of the internet, any web addresses or links contained in this book may have changed since publication and may no longer be valid. The views expressed in this work are solely those of the Author and do not necessarily reflect the views of the publisher, and the publisher hereby disclaims any responsibility of theirs.

The Author of this book does not dispense medical advice or prescribe the use of any technique as a form of treatment for physical, emotional or medical problems without the advice of a physician, either directly or indirectly. The intent of the Author is only to offer information of a general nature to help you in your quest for health and wellbeing.

In the event you use any of the information in this book for yourself, which is your constitutional right, the Author and publisher assume no responsibility for your actions.

Any people depicted in stock imagery provided by individual sources have been approved by that source and photographers.

Contents

Introduction p6

Chapter 1 – I would ask myself: 'Oh, why bother?' p13

Too hard

Too much temptation all around me Stress

I hate exercise Time to ditch excuses

So why bother?

Chapter 2 – As A Child p24

My love for food as a child

Working hard for pocket money to buy treats

Never dreamed of being over-weight

Chapter 3 – My basic Ingredients list to long-term weight-loss p38

Blood test

Proper Mindset

Water

Increase Energy

Exercise

Positive thinking

Patience and perseverance

Prebiotics (very important!)

Probiotics (Helps to cut down cravings for sugar & Keep your bowels regular)

    A bunch of veggies

A pinch of sugar

Weigh yourself once a week

Get enough sleep

Boost metabolism

Prayer and faith in God (Optional but it helped me the most)

Chapter 4 – Conclusion   p140

A summary of what we have learned

Introduction

First, I would like to mention that this book is not intended to diagnose or treat illnesses/diseases and must never take the place of professional advice. This is simply my own personal life experience and how I have dealt with obesity and finally reached my goal weight.

Please Note: I am not a nutritionist, dietitian or health care professional. I am simply just sharing my experience and hope to inspire as many as I can to live a healthier, happier life. Consult with your doctor before you decide to change your lifestyle and diet.

I do not guarantee any results of any kind. My 35-kg weight loss took me 15 months and a lot of daily hard work, focus & dedication.

You are probably thinking "Not another weight-loss book again! I have read so many and so far, none of them have helped". Before you decide to close the book, I am letting you know that there is hope for anyone that is genuinely willing to change his/her life for good and it can be done.

It took me 18 years to figure it out and learn from mistakes and if I can do it, anyone can. I decided to write about my experience so that others can learn from my mistakes and my experience over the years.

As the wise quote from John C. Maxwell reads:

"It's said that a wise person learns from his mistakes. A wiser one learns from others' mistakes. But the wisest person of all learns from other's successes."

— John C. Maxwell

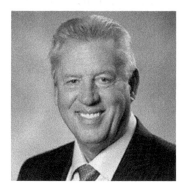

I believe that, just as the above quote states, you will learn from my mistakes, and from the success I have had in reaching my goal weight!

You probably scanned the table of contents and looked at my list of ingredients for natural weight-loss and thought "Well I already know all this, why should I waste time reading this book?"

Fair enough, you may already know that water is important in weight-loss along with patience, perseverance etc. I try to dig deeper into each ingredient and explain the benefits and write about my own experience.

I also write a bit about my childhood years and how food has always been precious to me (especially treats), they were quite rare in a communist country. Maybe you can relate to some of my experiences and learn from them.

English is my second language so expect this book to be written in simple English. I was born in Europe and only came to Australia when I was almost 9 years old; I did not even know one single English word.

Grade 1 and 3 months of grade 2 were studied back in Europe and when I came to Australia, they assessed me and placed me in grade 4 along with my twin sister.

I remember we were Being bullied every day because we did not know any English. We took part in special English sessions each week and slowly started to pick up the language.

We must have sounded funny trying to pronounce different words and repeating them over and over to remember them. Kids were laughing at us every day, but it did not stop us, we kept persevering. It was exciting – A new country – A new language!

This kind of brings me back to weight-loss. Nobody should ever give up on his/her dream to be healthy and fit. With patience and perseverance and the rest of the ingredients I list in this book, it can be achievable.

In Australia alone, over 50 percent of the population are overweight. Back when I was overweight it was encouraging for me to know that I was not alone in this struggle, more than half the population in Australia were going through my painful experience.

In May 2014, I decided to end this painful struggle once and for all. I started out on my final weight-loss journey and you can read all about my experience in '**My 18 Year Weight-loss Journey'** book.

I go through all my past failed attempts within the last 18 years, what hasn't worked, as well as what has worked for me. I share with you the <u>4 Key steps I needed to take</u> in addition to the basic foundation to natural weight-loss I write about in this book (My list of basic ingredients to natural weight-loss).

I truly hope to motivate, inspire you and all those out there that are faced with this challenge. I am living proof that we can do anything we set our mind to. We all have different challenges in life, different goals we want to reach and there are always obstacles along the way.

We must not allow obstacles to stop us. My mission is to encourage you to persevere and never let go of your dreams because you can do it. If I did it, anyone can!

I am not perfect. I have reached my goal weight but have also slipped off the wagon a few times. I have gained a few kilos here and there, but I always lose them to get back to my goal weight. I keep persevering and going forward. I never want to give up and go backwards to a life of pain, disease and misery.

In my book 'My 18 Year Weight-loss Journey' I write about how I have made that mistake in the past where I noticed I put on a few kg and stopped losing weight (even though I was doing everything right) so I would quit.

I would get discouraged, give up, turn to my previous unhealthy lifestyle and put on all the weight I had lost (20kg). I regretted that so much but also learned a good lesson from it and I will hold on to it with all my strength.

Finally, I want to thank God for the strength he gives me every passing moment. I owe him much more then I can ever repay back. He is my Hero.

Prayer and faith in him have brought me through some very tough times in my life and when the whole world seems to turn its back on me, God is forever there for me.

For those of you that do not believe in God or are not religious, you may have other ways where you find your strength so keep going with all you've got and believe you can do it.

Just a Tip:

If you want to make your journey easier, get your best friend or buddy to accompany you on your journey. This way you both build healthy habits and lose weight as well as be there for each other on days that are not so good.

Share my books with them, send them my author page or website so they can purchase my books and start this journey with you!

My website: **https://myweightlossjourneytips.com**

My Amazon author page: **http://www.amazon.com/author/irinadura**

Direct link to E-book version of this book:
https://www.amazon.com/gp/product/B0895B2GGB

Direct link to Paperback version of this book:

https://www.amazon.com/Natural-Weight-loss-Recipe-ingredients-naturally/dp/0648052079

Chapter 1 – I would ask myself: 'Oh, why bother?'

When I think back to when I started my weight-loss journey this question was lingering in my mind almost every day. I wanted to lose weight so bad, but I did not even dare to try anymore because I was afraid to fail yet again.

I would wake up tired, heavy and sore every morning and would start imagining 'oh…how good it would feel to weigh 65kg again, I would be light and not feel as tired and definitely sleep much better at night'.

But then followed the thought… 'oh…why bother? I already know I tried so many times and failed, it will be just a waste of time and energy' followed by painful disappointment.

When I would ask myself 'why bother?' the following excuses came to my mind:

Too hard

Yes, the weight-loss dream seemed so out of reach to me. I had struggled with obesity for 18 years, what makes me think that this time I will succeed? I have got to stop kidding myself and banish this dream from my mind once and for all.

But no…how can I settle for less than my dream of being healthy and fit? I had this constant battle inside of me and it was consuming me.

If only chocolate, ice-cream, chips and junk food never existed, it would have been so much easier for me but since they do exist, I must find a way to outsmart them all, but how?

I felt like junk food had me tied by a leash all day, every day, and I just could not escape. The more sugar I ate the more I craved it and I kept going around in circles and my weight-loss dream was drifting further and further away and out of reach.

Too much temptation all around me

Each time I would go out temptations where staring me right in the eye. I have a McDonalds just down the road and a Hungry Jacks just 5 minutes away.

In the little shopping centre where I buy groceries regularly there's a Baker's delight with mouth-watering chocolate croissants and Danish custard tarts which are my favourite.

I walk down a bit further in the mall and there's Fergusson Plarre Bakehouse with more mouth-watering goodies such as vanilla slice and my favourite whole-meal veggie pastie with the most amazing buttery flaky pastry I have ever tasted. Oh, and who can forget the passion fruit slice.

Time to get into the supermarket and I am bombarded with more temptations like iced doughnuts, freshly baked biscuits, chocolate, chips, muffins, ice- cream corn chips, freshly baked bread that smells divine and so on…

Stress

Everyone that knows me in person also knows that I am a stress head. I stress for everyone I know and worry about everyone and everything. This is the biggest obstacle when trying to lose weight because the more I stress the more comfort food I crave, so it is a never-ending cycle.

I figure why bother trying to lose weight? If stress stands in the way I have no chance. Sometimes my day starts off good and then I would turn on the TV and it happens to be the news.

I would see disturbing and sad things that happen to people around me and would start feeling sorry for them and worrying about them and everyone else that were affected. This sadness affects me deeply and so I would automatically head for my comfort food.

I hate exercise (then, not now)

I used to hate exercise with a passion! I hated the thought of getting all sweaty and showering and changing multiple times a day. I knew my muscles would hurt for a few days until I get used to the exercises. I also hated the thought of going to the gym or having to walk outside in cold, rain or in hot weather.

I have always feared exercise because of running out of breath and the stitches I would get in my stomach. I remember I used to get that at school when we were forced to run 2-3 times around the big oval each morning.

I had to learn the right way to approach exercise and make it enjoyable to the point where now I just don't feel good if I miss a day of exercise. I have lost 35kg (77 pounds) in 15 months just by walking and climbing the stairs in my house (and no, you don't have to climb stairs to lose weight, stairs was 20% and the 80% was walking).

Exercise doesn't have to be strenuous, painful and boring. I chose what was most comfortable for me and easiest on my body. If it was up to me, I would love to swim every day but so far nobody has been able to teach me how to swim.

They tried to teach me how to swim when I was in school, friends tried a few years ago, but to no avail. I just can't stand the thought of taking my feet off the ground and throwing myself into the deep water.

I must have gone through a horrible experience with deep water when I was little because we lived in a City by the sea. I remember grandma and grandpa taking us to the beach when I was little and I was very scared of the water.

In my book (My 18 Year Weight-loss Journey) I share how I started to finally enjoy exercise and look forward to it as well as how my first session was just 15 min because my body could not handle more.

I share how that did not stop me, how I persevered and built my exercise up to 1 and ½ hours each day (divided into 2 sessions). Once again, you don't have to exercise as much as I did, you do what is comfortable for you.

After I reached my goal, I cut down my exercising time to 40 min, 5 days a week. Some days if I did not feel well, I did not exercise. Also, if it is nice weather outside, I will go for a walk outside if my daughter or a friend joins me.

Time to ditch excuses!

I thought to myself that I must stop making excuses for my bad habits. It's time to ditch these obstacles that are keeping me captive and start taking responsibility for my actions; face my fear of exercise. My health is on the line here and if I don't do something about it soon, it will be too late.

What about you? Are you kept captive by excuses? Your excuses may be different. For example:

- I am not ready for change
- I do not want to give up my comfort zone
- If I lose weight, I will have to buy new clothes
- I do not want to exercise
- I do not have time, there are too many good series on Netflix

Whatever your excuses may be, get rid of them all. Your health matters the most and is priceless.

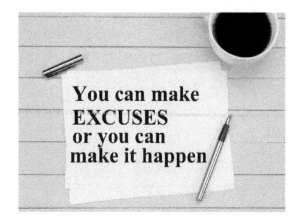

So why did I bother?

When I realized I am doing it for my health instead of just for looks and wear nice clothes I knew I had to make changes and ditch all excuses. I realized that health is the most important asset I can have, it is priceless. Without health, I will not be able to help others and be there for my loved ones.

The worst nightmare I can ever imagine of myself is being helpless in a wheelchair due to obesity and all the life-threatening diseases that come with it.

I started having visions of myself being morbidly obese, not being able to move around, being pushed around in a wheelchair and possibly with an amputated leg as a result of Diabetes. This really freaked me out and I did not want my kids to see me like that ever.

Take a few minutes to reflect on your excuses and write them down. Then write down all the reasons why you should bother to change your life. Writing and visualizing is powerful stuff.

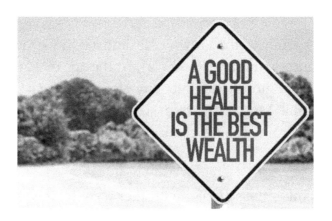

Chapter 2 – As A Child

I was born in a small town (Alexandria) in Eastern Europe in a communist country (Romania). At the age of 2, my parents decided to move to a larger city along the Black Sea called Constanta. Me and my twin sister had not started school yet but our brother being 4 years older had started school.

I remember the school my brother went to; it was just across the road from our house and I would often go and watch him play soccer with his friends after school finished at 12:30 PM.

On the long summer school holidays, we would often go to the small village where my grandparents lived and would spend the summer with them. It was around 6 hours' drive from Constanta.

I loved food for as long as I can remember. The beautiful dinner gatherings with my parents and often grandparents as well.

I remember each summer school holidays being taken to spend time with my grandparents and mum and dad would stay for a few nights before leaving us for the summer break and heading back to Constanta.

My sweetest memories are those around the dinner table where we would all enjoy delicious food and freshly baked bread from the wheat that my great grandfather and grandfather would grow on the field.

Jokes and laughter would fill the humble kitchen which was a small room adjoined to the back of the house and we would enter it from outside.

There was an old buffet style wall unit and it was light green. All the plates and cutlery would be kept there. The table was small, and we had a long bench along the back wall on which 4 of us would sit and on the other side of the table we had 4 wooden chairs.

In the corner, right next to the door there was the cook top that worked by wood fire only. The cooktop looked similar to the one in the picture below, only it was very old and tired:

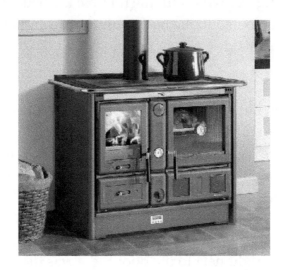

My great grandma would do most of the cooking and my grandma would make the bread. We would use the top of this cooker to toast bread slices. There was no such thing as a toaster back then in the humble village.

My love for food as a child

I simply loved food! It tasted nice, it brought us all together and mealtimes were my favourite part of the day. Having said that, I was not too keen on breakfast and ended up skipping breakfast almost every day.

For breakfast, it was fresh milk from our cow and sometimes sheep and goat milk too (we had all three and we also had chooks, a donkey, a dog and several homeless cats that my great grandma would feed).

My great grandpa would wake up early in the morning to milk the cow and then great grandma would boil it and then let it cool down. She would break pieces of bread in the milk and that was our breakfast.

I never liked milk of any kind so I could not eat it. Sometimes I would be starving, or it would be very cold winter mornings so I would eat but didn't like it at all – yuck!

By this time, we had started school and so my sister would have her breakfast and then we would walk to school which started at 7:30 am and finished at 12pm.

We would walk back home and great grandma would wait for us with lunch she had prepared. I remember they would all eat just breakfast and dinner and for us because we were kids, they would also feed us lunch.

Most of the times lunch would be Polenta with corn grown and harvested by us and milled at the local mill. The Polenta would be accompanied by country style potato chips and drizzled with a special garlic sauce that my great grandma would make, as well as fetta cheese and sometimes sunny side up eggs.

I cook this meal regularly here at home and each time I eat it, it brings back all those memories! Below is a shot of what this delicious meal looks like (missing the eggs this time):

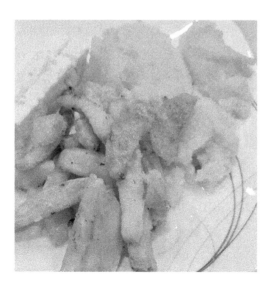

Polenta with home made oven chips, drizzled with garlic sauce.

Dinner was always the best because there was more variety. I would sit next to my twin sister on the bench along the wall and I particularly loved it when grandma would make fried eggs. We would have 2 each along with other food on our plate. I would eat quite fast while my sister was a very slow eater.

My favourite part was telling my sister 'Hey, look! There's a spider in that corner!' by the time she looked and tried to see a spider (which wasn't even there) I had already snatched a fried egg off her plate and eaten half of it... it was funny for the moment but then I did feel sorry for eating part of her food :(

She then would ask, 'where? I can't see it?' and then would go back to continue her eating and realize there's an egg missing from her plate. Then she would tell my great grandma (sad tone), 'grandma, she took an egg off my plate again and ate it'.

Great grandma would get mad at me and cook her another egg and if the chickens didn't lay enough eggs then my sister ended up having 1 less egg and that's when I really felt sorry for her.

If that was the case, I would often get a smack from my great grandma on my way out of the kitchen and be given extra chores to do as well…some days great grandma would chase me around the backyard with a stick however she never caught me.

Working hard for pocket money to buy treats

I loved food so much that I would wake up early with grandpa when he had to leave for work at 6am and work for pocket money. In winter, I would shovel snow to make footpaths to the front gate, the kitchen, the stables, the chooks, etc.

It used to snow heavily and by the morning sometimes we could not even open the door to get out of the house because snow was in the way. Sometimes the snow would pile up as high as 80cm.

In autumn, I used to sweep leaves in our yard and in the front yard to make it all look nice and clean. Sometimes I would scrub the really burnt pots and wash them to be ready for the next meal that needed to be cooked.

There was no such thing as 'non-stick' pots and pans and so food stuck to the pots and form a burnt layer.

Great grandma would first soak them in water then I would get an old spoon and scrape out as much as I could and then I would go in the back yard and dip a dish cloth in the sand and then use that to scrub the pots and pans, this is how it was done in the small humble village where I spent all my summer holidays.

I also had to clean out the chook pen, that was the worst! Dealing with the crazy chickens that were mad at me for disturbing them was not an easy task.

Apart from housework, my grandpa would pay me to learn each timetable and subtraction table off by heart. I was in grade 1 so I had to know them all off by heart, if not I would get hit with the ruler on my palms by the teacher at school. I would usually get 10 rulers on each palm.

Of course, she would hit me with the edge of the ruler. On top of the times tables the teacher would give us 1 new poem to learn off by heart each week and we had to stand up in class and say it in front of the whole class.

Grandpa was not rich, but he would pay me a little something for all my hard work, especially the moving of snow. Snow was very heavy, and I had to move it with a wooden shovel and throw it over out of the way to make a clear path.

I would save all the pennies he paid me and then buy treats that I loved from the canteen at school. Usually, it was soft caramels or chewing gum in the shape of cigarettes and wrapped in paper that looked like cigarettes.

Never dreamed of being overweight

As a child, I ate anything I liked and was skinny as a stick. I never even dreamed that I would ever have problems with weight. I used to see overweight people and did not understand what that is or why until later in life when I got to experience it for myself.

I must admit that as a child I was always active, always doing something and on the move. We did not even have a TV at home or at our grandparent's home which would encourage sitting down for hours.

My mum's auntie which lived across the road from my grandma had a black and white TV. I would sneak out of the house on some evenings to go and watch TV at her house. It's not like there was anything interesting on TV but I was just so fascinated by it since we didn't have a TV.

Being a communist country, they would control what was on TV and there was only 1 channel. I think the program on TV was only a few hours a day.

Other times I would sit down for 2-3 hours at a time was when I would knit with grandma and her friends. They taught me how to knit and I found it interesting and enjoyed it a lot.

The only thing is that whatever I was knitting never got longer then 15-20cm. I would knit a few rows and then make a mistake and then undo the whole thing and start again. I just could not stand to see that mistake.

When I knew a pattern well enough not to make mistakes, I would get sick of it and ask grandma to teach me a new one and so she did and again I would start and make mistakes, undo it all again and so on.

Great grandpa would look at me and say: "you know I've been waiting for that piece of work to get longer and waiting to see what will come of it but it's just not happening." I then explained how I keep undoing it because I make mistakes and then he would say: "It's ok, doing and undoing is good also, those who do that will always have something to do"….and he would laugh….

Other than my knitting episodes with grandma and her friends…I rarely sat down. The knitting was mostly in winter when it was very cold outside, and people didn't have work in the garden.

It was nice to sit by the heater and knit while everyone was catching up on the village gossip. In summer, everyone was busy outside in the garden.

I used to eat kilos of soft caramels all on my own and to not put on any weight was a miracle. I think it was because I was active and being a child, my metabolism worked at its best.

Below is a picture of me just a few months before coming to Australia. I was around 8 years old here and so happy as it was a special day.

We were dressed in special clothes and photographed so that our parents can see us. They had left the country 2 years before due to communism in our country. In my book 'My 18-year Weight-loss Journey' I write a bit about this experience and how it had affected me then, as well as later in life.

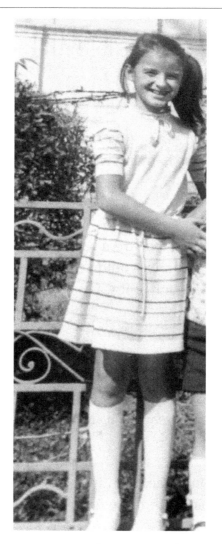

Me around 7 years old.

Chapter 3 – My Basic Ingredients to Long-Term Weight-loss

As I mentioned earlier, I never had a problem with my weight as a child. First time I remember putting on a kilo or two was when I was around 17.

Teenager, hormones and stress had to do a lot with it. I hardly ate sweets because mum wouldn't buy junk food, chocolates or ice-cream except only if it was a special occasion like a birthday.

Sometimes when we would travel by car from Melbourne to Sydney, we would stop for petrol and we would get a small chocolate or an ice- cream or a small bag of chips each.

We did not eat out either, we ate home- cooked meals every day. I think I was around 19 when I had my first McDonald's meal!

My real problem with weight gain started when I was pregnant with my first baby. As I share in 'My 18 Year Weight-loss Journey' book, I have struggled with weight for 18 years and finally decided to do something about it, the natural way, the way it's meant to be done for long-term results.

I have put together a list of ingredients needed for natural weight-loss to take place, the exact list that I had started following on my final attempt to reach my weight-loss goal.

This list of ingredients will lay the basic foundation to safe weight-loss and long-term results, as well as build daily healthy habits for life.

Here they are:

Blood Test

It may seem weird to you that I added 'blood test' as the #1 ingredient to the list and I have a good reason for it.

This is the very first thing that I did when I decided to lose weight back in May 2014. I struggled for 18 years, I would lose weight sometimes but would end up putting it back on and more. This time I was just feeling worse than ever.

I would get migraines almost every day, feel tired, stressed, depressed and my joints were aching so bad. I thought that something is very wrong with me and I must see my doctor.

The best way to know what was going on in my body was to get a blood test and that is exactly what I did.

Upon getting my results for my blood test I soon learned that my health was in bad shape. It opened my eyes to how sick I was and what this obesity was doing to me.

It was literally digging my early grave. It affected me to the point where I was ready to do anything it takes to save myself from this sinking hole.

I started asking myself: "What example am I setting for my children?" "I have to change, take responsibility for my actions and quit allowing food to control me."

As you can see, I put 'blood test' on top of my list of ingredients because it showed me what was really happening in my body, what junk food was really doing to me.

We do not have blood tests as often as we should and this is how disease creeps in slowly and takes us by surprise and in some cases, it is too late to do anything about it. I cannot stress enough how important this is.

Get a blood test done, know what is really going on in your body and then take action to heal your body and reverse the signs of sickness and disease.

And while you are at it, check your thyroid. Don't be content with just checking your TSH levels, make sure you specifically ask to get your T3 and T4 hormone levels checked. These will show if your Thyroid is underactive and causing havoc in your body.

Your thyroid controls hormones and metabolism so it is very important to have a healthy Thyroid! If your Thyroid isn't in top shape, your metabolism is not in top shape and weight-loss will be very slow and difficult.

Our body is a truly wonderful creation. It has the ability to heal itself but only if we are early enough and not leave it too late. Let natural food be your medicine and heal your body.

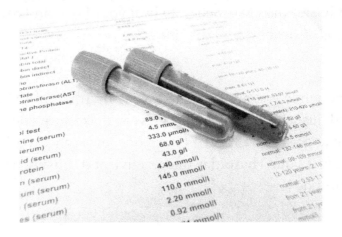

Positive mindset

OK, so for weight-loss to take place I needed to set up my mind. What is it that I want? How much do I want it? How much am I willing to do or give up for this to happen? Why do I want to do this? What is my ultimate goal? Who am I doing this for?

It's not until I started answering all these questions that I actually started doing something about it. I had to know the answers and my why and I explain all this in detail in my first book.

It wasn't enough to lose weight for the sake of looking good and wearing nice clothes, it was much deeper than that.

Grab a pen and write down any questions that come up in your mind about why you want to lose weight and get fit and then answer each question truthfully.

Keep this piece of information, it not only helps you to get to know yourself and what you are willing to do to finally make the change, but it will help you along your journey and keep you motivated.

Always remember, thoughts become actions and actions become habits. I have seen this working in my life for the past 2 years, the secret is to start paying attention to your thoughts.

Make sure they are thoughts that build you up and not drag you down. Fill your mind with uplifting, positive thoughts that will build healthy habits.

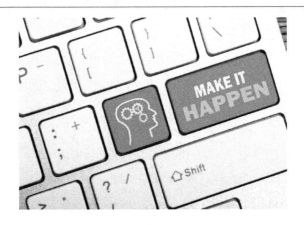

Water

I remember going a whole day with just 2-3 glasses of water especially in winter when I feel cold and the thought of drinking water would just give me goose bumps.

However, I have learned that water is very important and essential to weight-loss. It cleanses our body of waste matter and flushes out fat that is being melted away while we eat healthy food and exercise. It refreshes the brain and helps it to work at its best.

Water is the fountain of life; it helps to build more blood and oxygenates the cells. Water prevents constipation that can cause so many health problems including bowel cancer if not treated.

Our bodies can survive 3 days without food, but it cannot survive without water. This alone says so much about this awesome resource that God put on this earth for us. When I started thinking this way about water, I started drinking even if I wasn't thirsty or if it was cold outside.

I developed a daily habit of drinking water consistently throughout the day and 8 glasses minimum per day. I know people that drink soft drinks instead of water. That is pure disease, it is poison & creates acidity in the body and has absolutely no benefits.

Water helps flush the kidneys and keeps them healthy, it also helps in weight-loss because it cleanses the body of toxins. It is very important for hydration especially during and after exercise.

Water helps to keep your skin beautiful and hydrated. Water benefits our body in so many ways and we simply cannot survive without it. The quality of the water is <u>very important</u>, so I make sure that I always drink filtered water.

Are you a soft drink/fizzy drink addict? If you are addicted to soft drinks you will have to gradually reduce the amount of soft drink each day and replace it with water.

If you really don't like water then cut some lemon, orange (or any other fruit of your choice) and fill up a jug with water and infuse the fruit in it for a bit of flavour and aroma.

There is no excuse for not drinking at least 8 glasses of water daily. Write down every excuse that comes to mind about why you don't drink water and then really think about each one while at the same time thinking about the benefits of drinking water. The benefits will soon out-weigh the excuses and just cross them all out and get rid of them. Water is life and life is priceless.

On the other hand, don't overdo it. Drinking too much water can be bad for you as it can dilute and flush out important minerals from your body which can make you feel quite tired and sick so just keep that in mind.

Benefits of drinking water:

- Cleanses your body
- Boosts your metabolism
- Flushes out toxins and fat
- Cleanses the kidneys
- Essential to build healthy blood cells
- Hydrates your body
- Promotes beautiful skin

- Prevents wrinkles and fine lines
- Essential for optimal brain function
- Prevents constipation which can lead to life-threatening diseases

Make it a goal to drink at least 8 full glasses of water every day on top of any other drink or beverage. Stay away from soft drinks, energy drinks and fruit juices and only have it 1-2 times per week maximum.

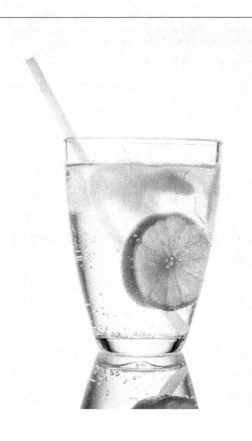

Increase Energy

I rely on energy every day. I need it to be able to complete my daily exercise sessions, do the housework, cooking, grocery shopping, work and of course be the best mum I can be for my kids. Without energy, I won't be able to function and complete my set tasks successfully.

So how do I increase my energy levels? I make sure I take the vitamins and minerals that my body needs in order to function properly (this is why a blood test is very important).

Two things that my blood test results showed were that I was very low in iron and vitamin D. I had to start taking iron and vitamin D supplements to build up healthy iron and vitamin D levels in my body. I have also had to have iron infusions as well. This has made a big difference in my energy levels.

I also drink my vegan protein shake daily which contains vitamins, minerals and amino acids. As I mention in 'My 18 Year Weight-loss Journey', I lost most of my extra weight without supplements.

However, towards the end of my journey the last pounds were hard to shift, that is when I added certain natural products that help boost my energy, mental focus and motivation as well as other benefits as well. Visit my website to check out the products I use and recommend at: https://www.myweightlossjourneytips.com

Energy boosting supplements give me energy that lasts throughout the day, unlike a cup of coffee where you get an instant kick of energy that dies down about an hour later and then you feel even more tired.

You end up going for another coffee because you need that energy kick again only to find that your energy dies out again.

Excess caffeine can put a lot of stress on your Adrenal glands and from then on you will end up with a whole lot of other health issues including inflammation and chronic fatigue.

What's worse is if you put a teaspoon of sugar in your coffee it's a disaster for weight-loss especially if you have it several times a day.

Coffee has benefits too (without sugar) and it's a great energy booster but for those like me that are sensitive to caffeine and milk, we must find healthier alternatives. For me it's green tea and other natural ingredients that help curb cravings for sweets and gives me energy.

Green tea also helps with anxiety. I feel that it refreshes my mind and sharpens my thinking. I get so much more done in a day when I drink green tea.

If I have a bad, unproductive day it is because I have forgotten to drink my tea or take my energy boosting supplements. It really is refreshing and revitalizing.

Having said that, Green tea does contain caffeine, but it is less than the caffeine content in black tea and in turn, black tea has a lot less caffeine than Coffee.

Green tea will give you a small caffeine boost but creates a gentler and steadier source of stimulation which can aid concentration.

Benefits of green tea

Cancer - Researchers believe that green tea can help kill cancerous cells due to the high levels of polyphenols it contains.

Heart Disease - Green tea contains catechins known to have protective effects on the cardiovascular system.

Working Memory – A research conducted in 2014 suggests that green tea can enhance our brain's cognitive functions, especially the working memory. It also suggested that it can help in the treatment of cognitive impairments with neuropsychiatric disorders such as dementia.

Weight-loss – Green tea may help with weight-loss in overweight and obese adults but since the weight-loss in the studies was minimal it cannot be ruled out as a clinical weight-loss contributor.

Other studies have found that green tea helps prevent dental cavities, stress, chronic fatigue, improving arthritis by reducing inflammation and helps treat skin conditions.

In my experience, it has helped because of the energy and boost it gives me and I am able to exercise daily. It also seems to clear my mind and I am able to make healthier choices.

Green tea may help fight prostate cancer. British researchers have scientifically proven that broccoli, turmeric, green tea and pomegranate help fight the most common cancer in men.

Green tea component upsets cancer cell metabolism.

A study reveals how an active component of green tea disrupts the metabolism of cancer cells in pancreatic cancer which explains its effect on reducing the risk of cancer and slowing down it's progression.

As with anything please consult with your doctor before you make any changes to your daily diet. Green tea as well as other energy boosting supplements are healthy but as with anything else it shouldn't be consumed in excess.

If you are sensitive, green tea along with other energy boosting supplements can cause insomnia if consumed after 2pm or if consumed in high quantities.

As I mentioned before, green tea helps with my anxiety, but it can also cause anxiety if you are overly sensitive to caffeine or drink green tea in large quantities.

Everyone is different so please consult with your doctor before you start drinking green tea or introduce any other energy boosting supplements and herbs into your diet.

Some herbs can interact with some medications so it's important to speak to your doctor especially if you are on any prescription medication.

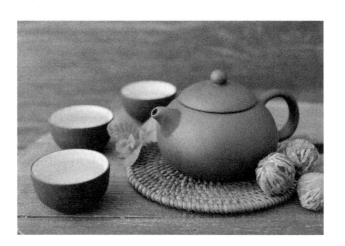

Other important ways to increase energy:

Get a blood test – find out what is really missing in your body. For me it was vitamin D and iron, both of which are energy boosters, if my vitamin D and iron levels are low, I will feel tired and lethargic.

Eat foods rich in iron. I choose iron from plants vs. iron from animals. Yes, iron from animals is better absorbed then iron from plant food and vegetarians may have lower iron stores then omnivores. Eating iron from plant food with vitamin C rich plant food will ensure the iron will be absorbed efficiently.

For vegetarians and vegans, it's important to note that *while they have lower stores of iron, they do not have higher rates of anaemia.* Researchers have found that many vegetarians' stores are 'low-normal,' but this does not mean less than ideal!

There's more evidence that says low-normal iron stores are beneficial: improved insulin function and lower rates of heart disease and cancer. Some of the best sources of iron in plant foods are:

Legumes: *Lentils, soybeans (non-GMO), tempeh, lima beans.*

Grains: *Quinoa, fortified cereals, brown rice, oatmeal*

Nuts and seeds: *Almonds, hazelnuts, cashews, pine nuts, pumpkin seeds, un- hulled sesame.*

Vegetables: *tomato sauce, Swiss chard, collard greens*

Other: *blackstrap molasses, prune juice*

Boost your B vitamins – B vitamins are great stress relievers also. When I'm stressed it uses up a lot of my energy and I start feeling tired. I have found that B vitamins give me energy and improves my mood.

As I mentioned before, I use the vegan protein shake as well as another supplement every day. These contain the B vitamins that the body needs daily to perform at it's best.

Eat complex carbohydrates such as:

Wholegrain breads and pastas (buckwheat, brown rice, whole wheat, oats, barley, quinoa).

NOTE: Be careful with wholegrain breads and pastas. Yes, they are healthy and contain healthy fibre for our body, but the body converts them into glucose which is sugar. I don't believe in leaving out whole- grains out of the diet because they contain beneficial nutrients for our body.

I make sure I eat wholegrains no more then 3-4 times per week and am super careful what I put on my bread. 99% of the time it's not the bread that packs on the fat, it is what I put on my bread such as fattening dips, margarine, processed cheese slices, nutella, jams etc.

For healthier alternatives switch to avocado and pure butter (healthy fats in small amounts). Instead of margarine just drizzle cold pressed olive oil on your bread, it is healthy and tasty too.

Instead of jam just cut up thin slices of fruit such as kiwi fruit, banana, strawberries and place on your toasted bread. A drizzle of natural honey on toast topped with thinly sliced strawberry slices and coconut cream can take the place of unhealthy desserts and it tastes yummy too.

Natural peanut butter without added sugar is also a healthy alternative for toast and you can drizzle a tiny bit of natural honey on top for natural sweetness.

Back in my country, bread was the most important food. We ate it at every meal even if we were having pasta, potatoes or rice. Because I grew up with bread at each meal it was challenging for me to cut down on bread.

I managed to cut down on bread because I understand the benefits of not eating bread at each meal or even every day. I noticed I felt better and that encouraged me.

As a child, I remember being hungry in between meals and the only available snack was bread. I would go and break a piece from the bread grandma made and would eat it on its own or sometimes with a piece of feta cheese which my grandma would make from fresh milk from our cows and sheep.

More Complex Carbohydrate Foods:

Lentils, kidney beans, chickpeas, split peas, soybeans (non-GMO). Fruits and vegetables such as: Potatoes (not fried), tomatoes, onions, okra, dill pickles, carrots, yams, strawberries, peas, radishes, beans, broccoli, spinach, green beans, zucchini, apples, pears, cucumbers, asparagus, grapefruit, prunes.

Complex Carbs: 2 Types of Fiber

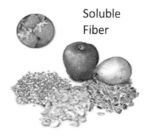
Soluble Fiber

Binds with cholesterol, preventing its GI absorption

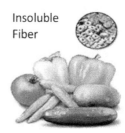
Insoluble Fiber

Adds bulk; stimulates "regularity"

These foods digest better because they are rich in natural fibre. They help with weight-loss because they keep you full for longer, as a result you will have less cravings (as long as you keep away from sugar as that is what sends your cravings through the roof). These natural foods if prepared the correct way (not fried), will keep your heart healthy.

For beans and lentils, I usually make soups or salads or just make bean burritos with red kidney beans. I keep all my cooking as close to nature as possible.

Even just boiling the beans and lentils in a vegetable broth for flavour would do. I then drain them and add a bit of olive oil and seasoning and accompany with some boiled eggs, Greek Yoghurt and a simple garden salad or cabbage and carrot salad and I have a tasty healthy meal.

I avoid frying and if I make a sauce or for example the beans for the bean burrito filling, I do not fry the onions in oil. I cook them in water and a few tablespoons of olive oil with a bit of veggie salt for flavour and sauté it with the lid on and then I add the rest of the ingredients and continue my recipe.

With spinach, I just cook it covered with lid on, with a bit of olive oil and salt and drain the juice and just serve it with poached eggs. Sometimes I add it on toast and sometimes on a bed of oven roasted asparagus and there I have another tasty, healthy meal full of vitamins, minerals and protein.

I just wash the asparagus and trim off the ends. I lay it on an oven tray lined with baking paper and drizzle extra virgin olive oil and garlic salt on top and bake it in the oven until lightly roasted and cooked.

Mushrooms are healthy and rich in B vitamins. I simply chop them to whatever size I feel like (sometimes chopped in half, sometimes whole, sometimes thinner slices) and place them in a large non-stick pot, drizzle with olive oil and veggie salt put the lid on and cook them for about 5 minutes. I then take the lid off and cook off the extra juice.

Sometimes I eat them just like that accompanied with sweet potato, potato or pumpkin mash and Greek yoghurt.

Other times I beat 2 eggs to which I add oregano and a bit of salt and pepper and pour them on top of the cooked mushrooms and let it set like a frittata and flip it on the other side and cook it. Again, another delicious, nutritious meal I can enjoy without feeling guilty.

Another favourite quick meal of mine is chopped mushrooms on a plate, topped with 1 chopped tomato, veggie salt to taste and about half cup of mozzarella or mozzarella cheese. I microwave it for 1 minute and enjoy. This can also be cooked in the oven.

As for sweet treats, I just eat green apple, pineapple, strawberries, blueberries, kiwi fruit, oranges, grapefruit. I enjoy a bit of chocolate or other sweets on the weekend. Bananas I try not to have every day but the other fruits I mentioned are all low-sugar fruits and they help to cleanse the liver and bowels.

A diet rich in vegetables has been shown to lower LDL cholesterol and help prevent against angina and heart attack by lowering blood pressure. Whole grains and legumes also help to protect the heart by lowering cardiovascular and coronary heart disease risk as well.

IMPORTANT

All carbohydrates (simple and complex) will be converted into glucose. That's why it's best to eat complex carbohydrates, they contain fibre which will help balance out the glucose and keep blood sugar at healthy levels.

It's important to eat smaller meals so that when the meal is converted into glucose it won't be overwhelming for the body.

Avoid simple carbohydrates, have it just as a treat a few times per week (2-3 times max for me). It contains no fibre, sends your blood sugar levels through the roof and won't keep you satisfied.

Simple carbs are: White flour, white bread, sugar, chocolate, candy, pastries, doughnuts, cookies, lollies, soft drinks, white pasta, white rice, croissants, Danish, cupcakes, pizza, noodles, fries, chips, potato crisps, white crackers, most cereals, etc.

✓ COMPLEX CARBS

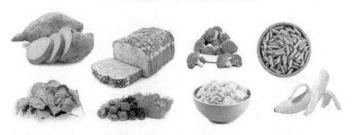

✗ SIMPLE CARBS

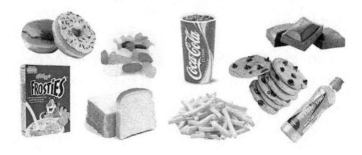

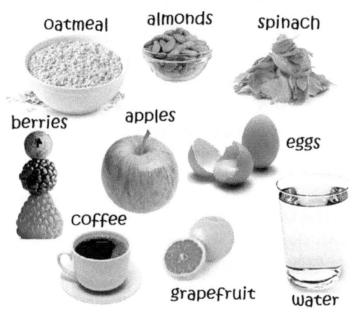

Get enough sleep (this is one of the ingredients on my list and I will get back to it later in this chapter).

Cut back on caffeine. It gives you a quick energy fix, but the energy will not last long, and you end up feeling more tired (especially if you have sugar in your coffee).

Coffee dehydrates your body and you would have to drink 2-3 glasses of water after a cup of coffee to replace lost fluids. It also creates a dependency and can cause anxiety and disrupt your sleep if you are sensitive to caffeine.

Here is what Goldstein of Harvard's Bringham and Women's Hospital in Boston had to say about coffee and its effects:

"…[Goldstein] found that people who drank coffee generally described themselves as sleepy in the mornings. That could be why they drink coffee, of course, but in fact what we find here is that when people stop using coffee, morning sleepiness doesn't get worse, it goes away."

Here we see that coffee can make us sleepy. Here's more to suggest that coffee contains a chemical to which the body reacts with the natural opposite which is sleep.

"People who keep on topping off their caffeine reserves throughout the day, however, will always have a substantial reservoir of the chemical in their bloodstreams: a prime condition for the body to redress its biochemical imbalance by boosting production of counter-caffeine chemicals. "

So, by drinking coffee we not only develop a tolerance to caffeine, but our body struggles to counter its presence in our system by making us even more sleepy.

The only way to stop this vicious cycle is to reduce caffeine intake. This however comes with unpleasant withdrawal symptoms as Goldstein says:

"…interruption in the caffeine supply can have severe and debilitating side effects: violent headaches, uncombatable drowsiness, and frequently depression."

The best way to make this a bit more pleasant is to replace coffee with green tea, it helps with anxiety and gives you sustained energy levels during the day just as I mentioned earlier.

I am not saying coffee is bad, it depends on each individual and how sensitive they are to coffee. I drink coffee mostly as a treat when I go out with friends.

Coffee is rich in antioxidants and has been proven to be healthy for the liver. For people that are sensitive to caffeine it can disrupt their sleep. We need quality sleep for our body to function at its best.

When I do drink coffee it's never later then 1pm. It's best to drink coffee without adding sugar to it as sugar is a chemical and it upsets the liver plus it's also addictive. The more you eat it the more you crave it. Switch to natural sweeteners such as stevia.

Growing research shows that coffee drinkers, compared to non-drinkers, are:

- Less likely to have type 2 diabetes, Parkinson's disease and dementia

- Have fewer cases of certain cancers, heart rhythm problems and strokes.

In case you were wondering, here's what a 240ml cup of coffee contains:

Vitamin B2 (Riboflavin): 11% of the RDA. **Vitamin B5 (Pantothenic Acid):** 6% of the RDA. **Vitamin B1 (Thiamin):** 2% of the R D A .

Vitamin B3 (Niacin): 2% of the R D A .

Folate: 1% of the RDA. **Manganese:** 3% of the RDA. **Potassium:** 3% of the RDA. **Magnesium:** 2% of the RDA. **Phosphorus:** 1% of the RDA.

Exercise daily
– this really gives me more energy and gives my brain a wake-up call. If you hate exercise don't worry, I also hated it with a passion.

If you haven't read my other book yet (My 18 Year Weight-loss Journey), get your copy and learn how I got past my fear of exercise and how I started exercising every day.

Reduce stress, forgive others, Forgive yourself. Find ways to reduce stress and <u>deal with anger right away.</u> If there's a strong will there is always a way. This is a must and very important.

Stress and anger use up so much of our energy and is toxic for our body. Find ways to reduce stress and let go of anger.

Stress can be caused by different circumstances. It can be your job, a major change or trauma in your life, losing a loved one, relationship problems, money problems, a friend or relative that has hurt you, raising babies and kids (as well as having the housework done, planning meals, doing the grocery shopping, paying bills), trying to lose weight, bullying, homework (for students) etc.

We all go through stressful times, but we must find ways to deal with stress or it will take hold of us and make us sick. When you are sick you can't function at your full potential.

Stress brings on anxiety, depression, heart problems, messes up your blood sugar, increases inflammation and feeds cancer cells.

If you find that stress has taken hold of you it's best to see a Psychologist. A Psychologist will help you sort through your problems one at a time and teach you ways to deal with everyday stress.

Stress also affects your Adrenal glands. It triggers them to pump out excess Cortisol which is the stress hormone. This causes pain and inflammation in the body and even more stress. It is a vicious cycle.

Start reducing stress by doing something for yourself each day, for example a hobby you love. Try to work on your hobby 15min, 2-3 times per day. Try going for a 30 min walk outside in the fresh air.

Start a 'Positive' Journal. Write down each day 3 positive things that have happened during the day. This will train your mind to think positive instead of dwelling on the negative.

Forgiveness sets you free.

Forgive easily and don't hold grudges, it will do you harm and poison your body. Do good to those that have hurt you and always have the strength to say sorry and make peace.

I personally like to live in peace and be at peace with everyone. I stay away from revenge and take it all to God, I know he takes care of everything.

If someone hates me or hurts my feelings, I just pray that God will give me power to forgive and have love and kindness towards the person/s involved. I feel liberated and free. I know that with God on my side I'm in the safest hands.

Prayer and the beautiful promises in the Bible are my only hope and strength in my everyday life. Why? Because I have experienced God's love and protection towards me and have seen the power of his promises being fulfilled in my life.

Sometimes it takes long, even years, but God always takes care of me and does that in his own time, his own way, and when he thinks it's best for me (lessons to be learned through trials).

This reminds me of the 18 years I have struggled to lose weight. I would have loved it to be instant just like a miracle, but God had a different plan for me.

When I was ready to allow him to take control (through daily prayer) and trust him fully, it was only then that he taught me lessons of patience, forgiveness and completely 'free' myself of any grudges I held on to.

He had to teach me lessons on my unhealthy eating habits and it wasn't until I understood that I needed a lifestyle change and the importance of 'eating to live' and turning back to nature that I truly started seeing results.

Beautiful promises like these gave me strength and hope every day:

"Come to me, all you who are weary and burdened, and I will give you rest". Matthew 11:28

"Cast your cares on the LORD and he will sustain you" Psalm 55:22

"Taste and see that the LORD is good; blessed is the one who takes refuge in him". Psalm 34:8

THE FIRST TO APOLOGIZE IS THE BRAVEST. THE FIRST TO FORGIVE IS THE STRONGEST. AND THE FIRST TO FORGET IS THE HAPPIEST...

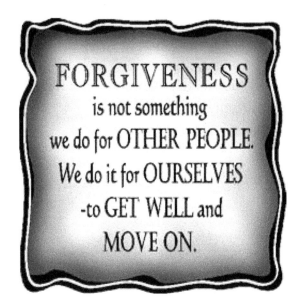

FORGIVENESS is not something we do for OTHER PEOPLE. We do it for OURSELVES -to GET WELL and MOVE ON.

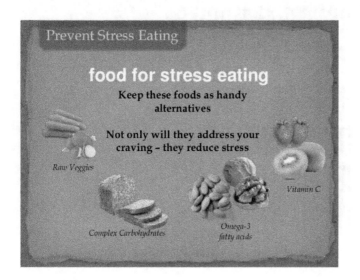

Some foods that reduce stress are raw veggies such as carrots, radishes. Vitamin C rich fruit,s such as strawberries, kiwi fruit, oranges.

Complex carbohydrates such as wholegrain bread. Omega 3 fatty acids such as walnuts and almonds.

Forgive yourself

Do not forget to forgive yourself and be kind to yourself whenever you end up disappointing yourself. I had to learn this lesson during my 18-year journey to lose weight. I was harsh on myself and hated myself for not being strong and always giving in to food.

Each time I would start a 'diet' I would give up after 2- 3 days and I would be so disappointed with myself and put myself down. I learned that it caused even more harm because I would turn to food for comfort.

Within my 15 months of losing 77 pounds, I wasn't perfect. I had days when I would eat unhealthy food or not drink at least 8 glasses of water and sometimes (rarely) I would miss my exercise session due to not feeling well or some other emergency came up.

If I allowed my 'old self' to come to the surface, I would beat myself up for all those 'shortcomings' and would get so upset to the point where I would say "oh what's the use…I keep failing, I may as well stop trying" and with that I would start eating unhealthy food and return to a life of pain and disease.

However, because of the strategy I had built and my renewed mindset, I did not allow myself to slip back. I would tell myself 'it's ok, I won't fall into discouragement, I will march on towards my goal. I need to be patient and forgiving towards myself'.

Exercise

I used to hate exercise with a passion because of the bad memories of exercise at school. It took me 18 years to start enjoying exercise and to my amazement, I look forward to it.

Before you close this book (just because I mentioned exercise) and you hate it as much as I did, please stay with me as I share with you how awesome exercise is for your body.

You probably already know the benefits of exercise but maybe you are like me and need to read something 10 x over to be convinced and start doing something about it once and for all: -)

We all tend to find the easy way out in life and one of those things is avoid exercise. I see it even when I go to the supermarket for grocery shopping. People are constantly fighting over the closest car parking space to the supermarket entry.

Even if there is an empty parking spot 30 meters away, they will still choose to waste an extra 5 minutes to wait just in case the space closer will be available.

Most people simply don't want to walk the extra few steps. Some are in a hurry; some don't want to walk more than they 'have to' and some park close just so they don't get wet if it rains.

It is so easy these days, we get in our car and go wherever we need to go. Back in the day people had to walk or ride a bike. Even if they took a bus or train, they had to walk to the station. Some were lucky to live close, but others had to walk a long way. It was not easy but it sure was healthy.

I look at my kids and see how easy they have it. We have always lived far from school, so I always had to drive them. Ever since they started school, I have driven them to school and from school. They have always been protected from the heat, rain, cold and wind.

Back in my day when I was a child I had to walk to school, it was a 20 min walk. Winter in Eastern Europe was harsh. I remember walking through snow and on ice. I would fall quite a few times by the time I got to school and would feel sore.

To make it worse the nasty boys at school would throw large snowballs at me and on the way home they would throw me in the ditch and cover me with snow…by the time I arrived home I was sore, tired and freezing.

At least I knew that my great grandma would be waiting for us with hot food. Oh, how nice was the food that my great grandma would prepare for me and my sister!

The taste of the delicious home-grown food and the warm wood terracotta heater would take the pain away and make me forget those harsh mean boys until the following day…

No wonder I never gained weight as a child. I was constantly on the move. Walking, helping with housework, yard work and when great grandpa wasn't around, I would take his bike and ride it through the village.

Nobody was allowed to touch his bike. He had no idea how many times I fell over and his bike fell against the dusty dirt roads. It was a bike for adults and my feet could hardly reach the pedals, but I really loved to ride a bike and didn't have one for my age.

When I came to Australia we were enrolled in school and it was about 20 min walk and so we walked to school and back. I didn't mind walking it was relaxing.

I started hating exercise when I was in grade 6 and our teacher forced the whole class to run around the oval 2-3 times every morning for that whole year. It was horrible, I felt like my lungs would explode and got stitches in my stomach.

When I started having problems with weight and was searching for a solution to lose weight, I kept being bombarded with the fact that I have to exercise.

I would get so mad and would think 'well I guess I'm destined to be overweight forever because there's no way I'm going to start running or doing aerobics.'

However, throughout the years I have been doing a lot of reading on exercise and how it helps our body in so many ways, not just weight-loss. When I started looking at it from that point of view, I suddenly had more reasons to exercise.

I also learned that I didn't need to take up strenuous exercise in order to benefit me. I have learned that brisk walking every day will be even more beneficial then running as well as gentle on my joints

I started walking and noticed how good I felt, how it clears my mind and drives my depression and anxiety away. I noticed improved digestion and over-all health, reduced blood sugar levels (as I was almost diagnosed with Diabetes), and improved blood pressure.

If I didn't have a treadmill, I wouldn't have made exercise a daily routine. Buying a treadmill has been the best investment in my health. I couldn't have done it if I had to go outdoors every day.

Don't get me wrong, I love walking in nature but only if the weather is perfect and I am accompanied by someone! I don't like to walk alone and in wind, rain and bad weather.

When I was a child, I didn't even know the benefits of walking or that it was good for me, it was a necessity. I remember that just to walk to the bus stop to get to the nearest town it was a 20 min walk.

If grandma wanted to go to a bigger city, then we had to take the train and it was about an hour walk and that included taking a shortcut through a forest and crossing a small creek.

Now that I know the benefits of exercise, I look for opportunities to fit in as much walking into my day as possible.

Even with the kids I started parking the car further away from school so that we can fit in at least a 20 min walk each day. At the shops, I park a bit further away just to get those few extra steps of walking.

If you are like me and hate the thought of exercise it's probably because every time you think of 'exercise' you imagine running and strenuous aerobics. It doesn't have to be like that.

Just start walking either outdoors or get a treadmill. You probably already have a treadmill shoved in a corner of your garage, start using it.

If you have sore feet or joints, don't let it stop you. Losing weight will take that extra weight off your feet and joints and will greatly reduce your pain so it's worth it.

Keep imagining the after results and benefits you get through exercise; that will motivate you to build daily healthy habits and stick to them.

Start slowly, even if it's just a 5 min walk at first. Do that for a week and the following week increase to 10 min and just before you know it you will find yourself walking 30+ minutes per day.

Walk at a comfortable pace, when you are used to it, increase by a point (on a treadmill), do that for 1-2 weeks and then increase again until you reach 'comfortable' brisk walking.

Walking will increase blood circulation to the joints and help with inflammation.

Believe it or not, walking prolongs life, it delays ageing, and it doesn't matter at what age you start walking, the same benefits apply.

Dr. Mercola even goes to say that by walking at least 20-25 minutes per day you can add 3-7 years to your life span. The trick is not to sit, especially more than 2 hours at a time.

Sitting gives way to diseases like diabetes, heart disease, cancer and other life-threatening diseases. Inactivity holds out a great big banner that says to sickness and disease: "You are very welcome here and can settle in for life".

Of course, there is a time for sitting and resting, we are humans and need rest, but these days we are way too sedentary, that's why our hospitals are struggling to meet the demand of providing hospital beds. Most of the patients suffer from obesity-related diseases.

Considering we use cars to get to where we need to go (sitting), and so many jobs are office/administration jobs, we need to fit in at least 30 minutes of walking per day if we want to drive away disease and live a longer healthier life. The trick is to break a sweat with each walk or exercise you choose to do.

Another problem is the time we spend watching TV, playing games on iPhones, iPads or just in front of the computer. This is why the younger generation is starting to lean towards obesity.

I was in India for a few days and the tour guide was telling us that more and more young kids in India are diagnosed with Diabetes.

She said that as a nation they eat very high carb and high fat foods as well as a lot of deep-fried food and sweets. Add to that the fact that we are not exercising enough, and you have the recipe to disease.

In my childhood days, I would come home from school, eat something in a hurry and go outside to play with the friends on my street. We would either race to see who gets first to the end of the street, play hide and seek or play tag (tiggy in Australia) etc.

Playing hide and seek outdoors involved walking and running as we would look for large shrubs, trees, fences, cars etc., to hide behind.

These days' kids can't wait to get home and play PSP, games on iPads, iPhones or just waste time on social media. All these activities are very unhealthy because it involves sitting for hours at a time.

If you have kids, please make sure they are doing at least 30 minutes of physical activity per day. Set a good example for them, teach them the benefits of exercise and how it prolongs life and prevents many diseases.

The good news is that you can watch TV while exercising. Get a treadmill and put it in the room where you usually watch TV and walk while you watch TV. You could do the same with an exercise bike as well.

You will burn at least 500 calories in an hour while walking at a comfortable pace. Top that with replacing a can of coke (or any other soft drink you are addicted to) with water, and you have suddenly subtracted 640 calories from your usual daily calorie intake!

Repeat daily, 6 days a week and you will reduce your calorie intake by 3,840 per week!

Think of all the ways you can fit in more walking into your day and write it down. This is a note I keep on my fridge to remind myself why I exercise daily.

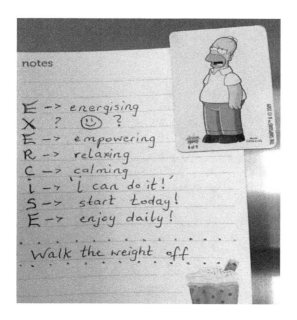

Positive Thinking

As I write about my experience in 'My 18 Year Weight-loss Journey' I mention how my negative thinking was a major reason of why I struggled with losing weight all those years.

This negative thinking fed my depression and anxiety. I had to change, do a lot of self-talk and replace negative thoughts with positive thoughts.

In order to achieve any goal in life we must take a positive approach, negativity will keep us from going forward. As soon as I started working on this issue that was holding me back, I started seeing results slowly but surely.

Take the time to identify all the negativity in your life, pay attention to your thoughts and find positive thoughts to replace the negative ones. There is positivity around us, but our unconscious mind automatically leads us into negative thinking.

As I was working on identifying and changing my negative thoughts, I saw improvement in other areas of my life, not just weight-loss.

Even right now as you are reading this page you might have had a negative thought about how this is too hard and how you will never be able to change your negative thoughts.

Write down your negative thought and then think of a positive one and train your mind to get rid of the negative and replace it with positive. For example:

'I won't get anywhere in life if I always allow myself to think that I can't change my bad habits or negative thinking. I can do it; anyone can do it if they really want to change'.

Or think about it this way: "If I don't think and do things differently, I can expect to be in the same place I am right now in a years' time." The question is, are you truly happy where you are at right now?

You must talk to yourself each time your mind tells you that you can't change your bad habits, or a negative thought comes to your mind. Keep doing this, practice it daily and it will soon become a habit, a routine.

Write each negative thought down and then under it write 'I will replace this with…' and write down the positive thought you will replace it with.

Please, never give up for your health' sake and your loved ones. You can do this. Negativity keeps us captive; it keeps us tied up in a world of pain, sickness and loneliness, let's not let it rule us and our lives.

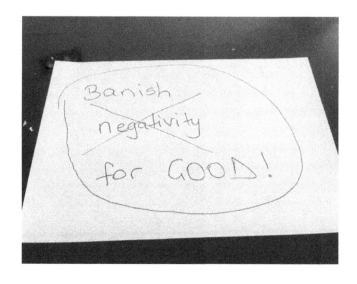

Patience and Perseverance

Once again, lack of patience has kept me from reaching my goal all those years. I would start a healthy lifestyle and would see how long it takes to lose a kilo and would give up because I didn't have the patience.

But what did I achieve by being impatient? I set myself up for danger and premature death due to all the diseases I was facing due to my unhealthy lifestyle.

You probably gathered from the Introduction section of this book that I love God and I owe him more than I can ever repay back for the strength he gives me every day.

I love the Bible and I hold so many Bible verses close to my heart because they strengthen and encourage me in my daily life. (If you are not a Christian, feel free to skip these few paragraphs.)

<u>There are many verses about patience and here are a few:</u>

'Be joyful in hope, patient in affliction, faithful in prayer.'
Romans 12:1

'But if we hope for what we do not yet have, we wait for it patiently.' Romans 8:25

'Wait for the Lord; be strong and take heart and wait for the Lord.' Psalm 27:14

All these verses give me hope, they assure me that if I trust in God, tell him about my goals and ask for his strength and help, he will help me providing I have patience to overcome obstacles along the way and am willing to take action.

He will help me if my goals are according to his will. Of course, being healthy and happy is God's will for all of us and so I knew that by asking God to help me in my goal to lose weight and change my bad habits, he would be more than willing to help me.

I remember all the times I am impatient and do things in a hurry, it always turns out bad and I end up telling myself "well I wish I was more patient".

The result of 'impatience' in my experience leads to having to do things all over again and waste precious time. I have learned to hold onto patience because it brings much better results and saves me time and frustration. Patience really is a virtue.

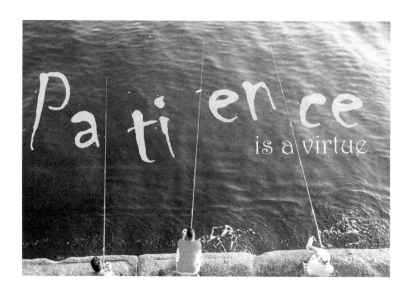

A bunch of veggies

It is utterly important that we feed our bodies with healthy food and I'm a strong believer in 'you are what you eat'. To me it makes sense to eat foods that are rich in nutrients, vitamins, living enzymes and are as close to nature as possible.

Veggies are full of all these things and are vibrant in colour like deep green, red, yellow, orange, light green, white etc. Veggies help to build healthy blood that helps to renew and rejuvenate our cells and feed them with renewed life.

Our cells renew between 2 days to as much as 8 years and some don't renew for a lifetime. Just like the following chart shows:

cell type	turnover time	BNID
small intestine epithelium	2-4 days	107812, 109231
stomach	2-9 days	101940
blood Neutrophils	1-5 days	101940
white blood cells Eosinophils	2-5 days	109901, 109902
gastrointestinal colon crypt cells	3-4 days	107812
cervix	6 days	110321
lungs alveoli	8 days	101940
tongue taste buds (rat)	10 days	111427
platelets	10 days	111407, 111408
bone osteoclasts	2 weeks	109906
intestine Paneth cells	20 days	107812
skin epidermis cells	10-30 days	109214, 109215
pancreas beta cells (rat)	20-50 days	109228
blood B cells (mouse)	4-7 weeks	107910
trachea	1-2 months	101940
hematopoietic stem cells	2 months	109232
sperm (male gametes)	2 months	110319, 110320
bone osteoblasts	3 months	109907
red blood cells	4 months	101706, 107875
liver hepatocyte cells	0.5-1 year	109233
fat cells	8 years	103455
cardiomyocytes	0.5-10% per year	107076, 107077, 107078
central nervous system	life time	101940
skeleton	10% per year	109908
lens cells	life time	109840
oocytes (female gametes)	life time	111451

So, as you can see it is very important what we eat because the blood that runs through our veins and heart is the very blood that feeds our every cell and renews it.

If our blood is healthy then our cells and organs are healthy, and we will feel healthy and energized.

Now imagine if our blood is built entirely from soft-drinks (refined sugar is a chemical), chocolates (more chemicals), white bread/white flour products (acidic environment for our bodies and feeds cancer cells), Meat (most of it is very acidic and especially red meat is linked to bowel cancer), Alcohol/beer (linked to liver cirrhosis, slowly but surely kills the liver), smoking (introduces carcinogens substances into the blood that impacts all cells in the body by distribution through the oxygenated blood).

I surely wouldn't want this kind of blood running through my veins, and neither would you!

Take a good look at the images below and ask yourself if it's worth feeding your body with foods and substances that damage your delicate cells and vital organs?

You know I often think about how we see so many sick people around us and dying in hospital of lung cancer, bowel cancer, liver cancer, Diabetes... and the first thing we ask ourselves is:

"Why does God allow this? Why is he so heartless? Doesn't he think of all the loved ones that are left behind?"

Well, it's not God's fault. It is our own doing. It is the bad choices we make, and each bad choice comes with consequences. He created the perfect drink and food for us: water, natural fruits, veggies, nuts and seeds, pulses (beans, lentils, chickpeas, soya beans), grains, all perfectly balanced with nutrients, vitamins and natural sugar.

Many times babies are born sick right from their mother's womb. Agan, first thing we do is blame God. Of course, that' what we do best, put the blame on someone else.

But do we ever think of the mother of the baby? What was her diet like? What about the baby's father? What about the parents of the mother's baby? What health problems did they have that their daughter carried on and passed on to her baby? And so on…

It was humans that came up with chocolate, soft drinks, refined flour, sugar, candy, Vodka/alcohol, drugs, cigarettes, genetically modified grains, fake cheese, and so much more.

God created water for refreshing and hydrating our entire body but when greed for money came into the picture humans came up with all kinds of addicting foods, beverages, fast food etc.

These greedy people knew that once they create a certain food/beverage/substance to the point where it's addictive, people will keep coming back for more which means more money for them.

If you find it hard eating greens and all the different veggies every day, there is an easier way for those of you that have no time to prepare your greens and veggies every day.

You can purchase high quality greens in powder or capsule form from your local vitamin store or search for good quality greens in powder or capsule form online. I use it myself and add it to my protein shake.

I am not a fanatic. I still eat chocolate, ice-cream, chips, pizza but only as a treat around 2-3 times per week. Before I used to eat chocolate and junk every day.

Look at the images below and ask yourself: 'Is it worth it?' Is it worth eating junk, drinking alcohol, soft drinks, smoking…just to get the results you see in the following images?

Write down all your current bad habits and why you should change your life starting TODAY.

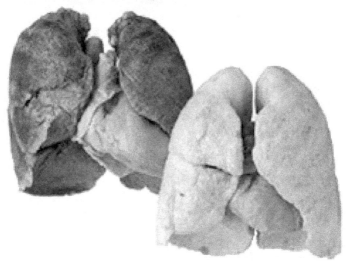

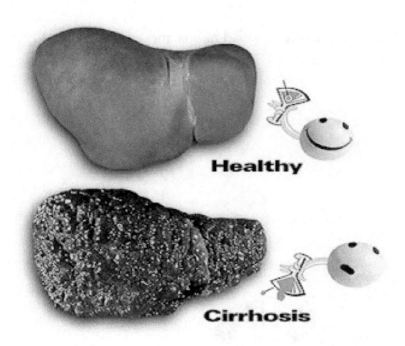

A pinch of sugar

Sugar gets blamed a lot for most diseases around us today, but sugar is necessary for our health and all the cells in our body need glucose to function. That's why I added 'A pinch of sugar' to my list of ingredients for natural weight-loss.

As I mentioned earlier carbohydrates contain sugar which the body converts into glucose. The problem is the 'added sugar' which is hard to keep track of because food labels only list information on 'total sugars' per serving.

For this reason it's best to eat as natural as possible and avoid packaged foods, white flour products (simple carbs), ready-cooked meals in the freezer section, sweet biscuits, packaged snacks, cakes, sweets, etc.

Cook most of the food yourself and keep it as simple and as close to natural as possible. In future, companies may be forced to list the amount of 'added sugar' to their ingredients list.

Banning chocolate and sweets out of my diet forever is not something that appeals to me. I have done that before when I attempted to lose weight and I gave up in a few days because I felt I was being punished for life.

If we never knew of chocolate, cakes, ice-cream then it would be a whole different story, we would not be in the mess we are now in the first place. Now that it's here, for those of us that love it, we can enjoy it as a treat only and in small quantities.

Those that are strong enough to totally get rid of 'added sugar' in their diet, I applaud them, I admire them.

I think it's important to have a treat every now and then as long as it's not every day. I know that during the week I must be good, make good choices, exercise daily and on the weekend, I can enjoy a bit of chocolate and cake as a reward.

Having sweets on the weekend means that during the week I give my liver a rest and a chance to cleanse itself.

We've known for decades that alcohol is responsible for liver cirrhosis, but we hear of more and more people dying from liver cirrhosis who don't even drink alcohol.

The answer to that is excess sugar and 'added sugar' in our daily diet. It is toxic for our liver and when consumed in large amounts (daily or even every second day) we are destroying our liver.

The liver has the capability to heal itself but as soon as it gets to the cirrhosis stage it is too late. We have the power to stop that from happening.

We must say no to 'added sugar' and only eat it (or drink it) as a treat in small quantities. Sugar is also acidic; it creates an acidic environment in our body and we know that cancer cells thrive in an acidic environment.

I have noticed that if I eat sugar during the week, (even if I exercise and watch my calorie intake), I won't lose enough weight at the end of the week because it blocks my body's ability to burn fat and function at its best.

Sugar is toxic for the liver and that is the reason why my weight-loss efforts are in vain when I consume sugar. I put sugar on this ingredient list because it's important to allow myself a little treat at the end of the week.

If I tell myself I will never have sugar, I will feel punished, get discouraged and give up on all the healthy habits I've built and implemented during the week. As a result of that I will return to my unhealthy lifestyle daily and put on all the weight I have lost.

If you love chocolate and sweets like I do then this ingredient is important to your long-term success, a pinch of sugar (chocolate, ice-cream, cake) only as a treat and stay away from it during the week.

I drink tea daily and don't put sugar in it. If you drink tea or coffee daily, you will have to leave out the sugar as it blocks your body and upsets your liver (which is responsible for the metabolism of fats).

The liver is the biggest fat burner in our body. It makes sense to eat foods that the liver loves and avoid foods that upset the liver.

Foods that your Liver loves

Your liver absolutely loves cruciferous vegetables such as:

Broccoli, Cauliflour, Kale, Brussel Sprouts, Cabbage, Dandelion leaves and herbs. It also loves Green tea, Milk Thistle and Turmeric herbs and Dandelion root tea.

Eliminate alcohol & Sugary foods. Reduce the amount of grains and grain products in your diet such as pasta and bread (especially refined/white).

Try to buy organic as much as you can as it reduces the amount of chemicals and pesticides on your fruits and veggies.

Also get rid of household cleaning products loaded with chemicals. These really upset your liver. I have switched my regular household cleaning products and laundry products to natural and safer products. Since I have made the switch, the severity and intensity of my migraines have been reduced to almost none.

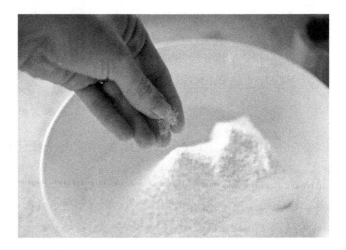

Weigh Yourself Once a Week

This is VERY important (in my experience). Weighing myself helped me face reality. At the end of each week if I wasn't happy with the results on the scales, I looked back at the whole week, looked closer at the food choices I made and made positive changes.

Sometimes I did everything right and I had to understand that I needed to be patient with my body because each week is different and certain changes take place in my body. This is where 'patience' comes in very handy and I am glad I persevered and didn't give up.

I don't recommend weighing yourself more often, once a week is enough and it makes you aware of your progress. If you are happy with the results, keep doing what you are doing and if not then re-evaluate your week and see where you might have slipped.

We are humans and we all fall off the wagon sometimes, the important thing is to pick ourselves up and keep going forward. Discouragement and 'giving up' should never even be considered.

I keep hearing people all the time to ditch the scales and start measuring. I don't really agree with it, weighing really helped me on my journey, it showed me reality, seeing 100.1kg on my scales was what opened my eyes to how overweight I was.

I also took measurements as well and my numbers changed on the scales as well as on paper.

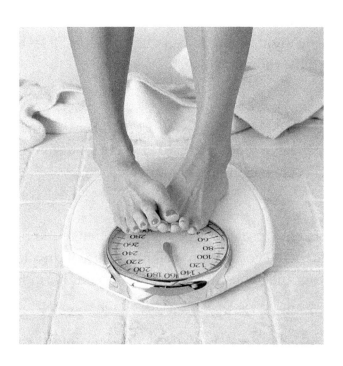

Get enough sleep

Once again, I will write from my own experience. Whenever I have a late night (going to bed after 10:30pm), I feel grumpy and tired the following day.

Not only that, I also crave comfort food because my body is tired and craves foods that will give me an instant energy boost: chocolate being first on my list.

Scientists at Uppsala University in Sweden found that lack of sleep can make you put on weight because it drastically slows down your metabolism and messes up your hormones.

Lack of sleep has negative effects on your mind. You will struggle at problem solving and dealing with everyday stress including making good decisions and healthy choices.

Lack of sleep can also suppress your immune system making you more vulnerable to infections. A study in 2009 found that sleeping less than 7 hours per night increased the risk of catching a cold.

Sleep makes you quicker and sharper, which means you will have more energy to exercise and be more active. Adequate sleep will also help your memory too.

A study has found that people who sleep less than 6 hours per night for 2 weeks, scored far worse in memory tests then those who slept 8 hours.

If going to bed late is a habit it is going to be a bit tricky to start going to bed early. The easiest way to train your body to go to sleep early is to start gradually.

If you go to bed at 12 am for example, then start by going to bed at 11:30 pm. On the following night at 11pm and so on until you get to 9pm.

Drink a warm cup of chamomile tea about an hour before you go to bed. It helps to relax your body and mind so you can fall asleep easier. Good quality magnesium powder helps as well.

Avoid a computer/iPad screen and playing games at least an hour before bedtime. Avoid caffeine after 2pm especially if you are sensitive to caffeine.

The trick is to get at least 2 hours of sleep **before** midnight. Sleep won't be beneficial to you if you don't get at least 2 hours of sleep before midnight. You can sleep 10 hours after midnight and still feel tired the following day.

In an article 'Rest and Sleep - Essential for Health' Dr. Lawrence Wilson suggests that it's best to go to sleep between 8-9 PM every night.

He writes that the hours before midnight are far more valuable for rejuvenation then those after midnight. He also writes that the hours before midnight are less conductive because the energy of the earth has shifted and the new day is starting. This brings a crescendo of solar energy that interferes with sleep, to a degree.

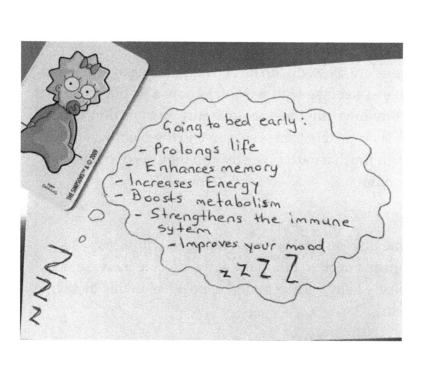

Boost Metabolism

Some of us are blessed with an active metabolism and never ever have to struggle with weight. I know a lot of people that can eat anything, anytime, any quantity and just don't put on weight. Their metabolism is so active to the point where they don't even finish a meal properly and they need to hurry to the bathroom.

As for me unfortunately, I wasn't blessed with a fast metabolism. I need to put in the extra effort to increase my metabolism. I always like to find a 'positive' in this by saying to myself:

'It's ok, it means I have to work a bit harder to increase my metabolism by adapting a healthy life-style and choosing metabolism-boosting foods – all of which will have long-term health benefits and will be a blessing to me'.

The good news is that it can be done naturally. I have already mentioned some natural ways to increase metabolism in the list of natural weight-loss ingredients above, such as:

Water - Drinking water can boost your body's ability to burn fat. A study published in the Journal of Clinical Endocrinology and Metabolism found that drinking water (about 17oz) increases metabolic rate by 30 percent in healthy men and women.

Exercise – Exercise will help boost your metabolism as long as you exercise for at least 40 min and break a sweat. Weightlifting is the best metabolism booster but I'm pretty happy with brisk walking, it has given me great results.

Muscle cells need a lot of energy, which means they burn a lot of calories. If weightlifting appeals to you then go for it! I may learn to embrace it as time goes by ☐

Just a word of warning: Just because you have burned 500 calories within 45 min of exercise, it doesn't mean you have to go crazy on food after your exercise session.

In the end, exercise is just a boost in weight-loss, the main contributor to weight-loss is what you feed your body with.

Exercise boosts your metabolism while you are exercising, and you will burn fat for about 15-30 minutes after your exercise session (depending on the intensity of the work-out).

Sleep - Sleep plays a vital role in regulating metabolism and appetite. When you are sleep deprived, your metabolic system will be out of balance which will affect the choices you make when it comes to your daily diet.

Teenagers who don't get enough sleep will crave more carbohydrates. Inadequate sleep is the risk factor for obesity in young adults.

Chronic sleep deprivation means you are getting less than 8 hours of sleep per night and it is associated with increasing your BMI (Body Mass Index).

A study conducted in the 'Wiscounsin Sleep Cohort Study' of 1024 patients showed that the shorter sleep durations the more reduced levels of leptin and elevated levels of Ghrelin.

- Leptin is a hormone that inhibits appetite and increases energy expenditure.
- Ghrelin is a hormone that increases appetite and reduces energy expenditure.

In another study that followed 70,000 women over a period of 16 years, showed that there was a significant increase in body weight in those who slept 5 hours or less compared to those who slept 7-8 hours.

As sleep time decreased over time from the 1950s to 2000s from around 8.5 hours to 6.5 hours, there has been an increase in obesity from about 10% to about 23%.

<u>Metabolism Boosting Supplements</u> – There are several metabolisms boosting supplements available on the market and they will give you that extra boost you need in losing weight however there is a danger in using weight-loss supplements.

From personal experience, I found that whenever I used weight-loss supplements I kind of lost track of my healthy habits because I was relying on the supplements to do the hard work for me and as a result I returned to my unhealthy habits and didn't lose any weight.

<u>Supplements can help but only… **and I really mean it**… ONLY if you are already implementing all the ingredients to basic weight-loss in this book in your daily life along with mindset, focus and determination as well as the strategy and steps I mention in</u> **My 18 Year Weight-loss Journey book.**

ONLY then you can add a safe natural metabolism boosting or fat burning supplement to your daily weight-loss routine just as an added bonus on top of the healthy ingredients to natural weight-loss mentioned in this book and the strategy and steps I mention in 'My 18 Year Weight-loss Journey' book.

I will always keep in mind that a 'miracle pill' for weight-loss will never exist and hard work, focus, determination and smart strategies are needed to reach my weight-loss goals.

I kept searching for and waiting for a miracle pill all those wasted years and never found it. It wasn't until I took care of my mindset, developed a daily strategy and took action that I finally started seeing positive results.

Through my 18 years of struggling to lose weight, I had to learn the hard way that supplements will never ever work for me unless I change my lifestyle and adapt to healthy habits daily.

As a result, I have lost 77 pounds within 15 months and am sharing with you my basic ingredients to form a foundation to natural weight-loss and a lifetime of healthy habits.

Yes, natural weight-loss supplements will make your journey easier and speed up the process BUT you must accompany them with the steps and strategies that I share in both my books.

You can check out my website as sometimes I share natural products that I personally use. They have really helped me on my journey: **www.myweightlossjourneytips.com**

Always remember, healthy lifestyle first: switch to foods that boost metabolism, exercise daily, drink at least 8 glasses of filtered water daily, get adequate sleep.

Once you implement these steps into your daily life you can add a safe, natural metabolism-boosting supplement as a helping hand to your already healthy foundation you have laid for natural, safe weight-loss.

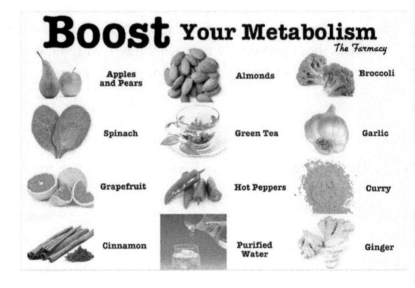

Prayer and Faith in God (Optional but has helped me the most)

If you don't believe in God feel free to skip this part :-) Personally, this has been my most important and most powerful ingredient in my final weight-loss journey and in my daily life in general. Without this, I honestly couldn't have reached my goal.

When I reach a point in my life where I feel that I can't accomplish something or reach an important goal, my immediate 'go-to' is God.

Ever since I can remember as a little child with any little problems I had, I have always gone to God for help. For you to understand why God is so important to me, I will tell you how I started to know God and how I grew to love and trust him as much as I do.

My relationship with God and Jesus started as early as I was able to understand stories that my grandma would tell me. She would tell me about how we each have our own guardian angel that watches over us every second and keeps us safe from any danger.

I would ask what heaven will be like and she would tell me how there would be no tears, pain, sickness, diseases, evil of any kind and death. That really raised curiosity in me to find out more about this wonderful place called heaven.

I would ask her all kinds of questions and would be all eyes and ears to find out the answers. She would tell me that there will be no night in heaven (I was always scared at night and found it hard to fall asleep).

She would tell me that the streets would be of gold and that the lion will sit with the lamb and there would be perfect peace and harmony.

I loved hearing about heaven and held it all dear to my heart and I would dream at night that I was in heaven and there were angels all around me and it was just the most beautiful place I had ever seen.

She would tell me Bible stories and parables that Jesus told, and she would point out the lessons that are to be learned from all the stories throughout the Bible and the life of Jesus.

She would teach me to pray to God every day and tell me that even if I don't see him, he hears me and even knows all my thoughts and the number of hairs on my head.

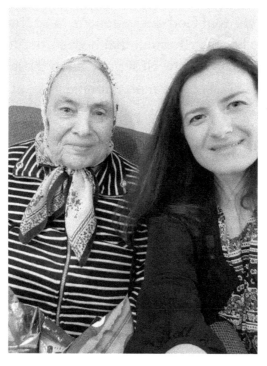

Me and my precious grandma Maria

That was so interesting to me. If he knows the exact number of hairs on my head then he must love me a lot and care about me, I thought. I even remember trying to count each strand of hair and gave up quite soon of course...

Sometimes I would see sad things happen to people that were close to God and loved him and as I grew older. My grandma explained to me that God does allow us to go through trials and hardship because through that he tests our love for him and faith in him. We draw closer to God in those circumstances, we become more humble, patient and better human beings.

I view trials and hard times as rain and storm. Just like flowers grow when it rains, we also grow through the 'rainy' periods of our lives.

Just like gold is refined through fire, so are we humans refined and cleansed through tough times and hardship that we go through but only if we remain close to God and never depart from him.

I began to understand that most of the time we bring trials and sickness upon ourselves because we make the wrong choices and consequences follow.

As humans, we can sometimes be very stubborn and only learn from mistakes that often hurt so much. I have seen this in my own children. I tell them "don't do this or that, you will get hurt" and yet they still do it and will only learn when it hurts them bad enough.

In the 18 years of trying to lose weight I failed to put the matter into God's hands and ask him to help me.

I thought this is not a matter to go to God with and that I already knew what I had to do. I just had to go on a diet and exercise. However, no matter how hard I tried, nothing worked.

I had to learn to finally realize that in my own power I can do nothing, I needed to go to God, ask him for strength, healing, patience, wisdom to make the right choices and a clear mind to be able to set up my mind and form a strong daily mindset.

I finally prayed to him when I couldn't take it on my own anymore. The burden was too heavy for me to bear. I knew the beautiful promise Jesus left for me when he was on this earth, he said:

"Come unto me all you that are heavy burdened and I will give you rest".

Here he invites me to leave all my burdens at his feet, everything that makes me so tired and fill me with anxiety and worries and he will carry it for me and give me rest.

I thought "Why am I resisting his offer to help me? It's free! Why am I struggling on my own when he is eagerly waiting to help me?"

So just before starting my final weight-loss journey I said a very heart-felt and emotional prayer to God. I was literally talking to him just like a child talks to his/her parents and tells them his/her problems.

For children to be able to do that it takes trust and the knowledge that they can actually help with his/her problems and they realize that they can no longer solve their problem on their own and they need help.

This is exactly what happened to me. I have learned that God is my father and I am his child and he is waiting with open and loving arms to help me.

He wants me to learn that I depend on him every single moment of my life. I have finally learned it and so I told him I am giving him this huge 'weight-loss' burden that I can't bear on my own any longer.

I came to him with all my pain and sicknesses that obesity had plagued me with. I told him that he has the power to heal me and I trust in him fully.

Just as Jesus healed the lepers, raised the dead and gave hope to the hopeless, he can do the same for me 2020+ years later. His power and love for me are unchanged and he is ready to help and heal anyone that loves him truly and trusts him fully.

I ask God's help in other areas of my life especially for the patience and wisdom I need to raise my kids in the way that he would want me to.

I put my life and the life of my kids, relatives, friends and loved ones into God's hands. I know that if we are in his hands, we are safe and truly loved.

Yes, we can be taken through trials, but it is OK as I know God is teaching us valuable lessons and drawing us closer to him, in the end we will be safe and blessed under his wings.

Once I learned to live my life this way, I have eliminated so much anxiety, worry and stress from my life and replaced it with peace and trust in my father in heaven.

"Come to me, all you who are weary and burdened, and I will give you rest". Matthew 11:28

"LORD my God, I called to you for help, and you healed me." Psalm 30:2

"Jesus went through all the towns and villages, teaching in their synagogues, proclaiming the good news of the kingdom and healing every disease and sickness." Matthew 9:35

As you can see, these are such beautiful promises full of hope and love. I have learned to never underestimate the power of faith in God and prayer. I have seen it work in my life and so many other people's lives.

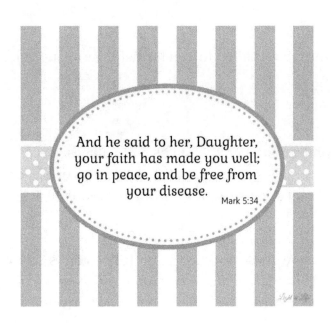

> I am the Lord who heals you.
>
> Exodus 15:26

www.WhatWomenShouldKnow.org

Chapter 4 - Conclusion

OK, we have gone over my basic ingredients list to safe natural weight-loss. I say 'basic' because in my book "**My 18 Year Weight-loss Journey**" I go a bit deeper into Mindset and a few other important steps needed for long-term success.

A summary of what we have learned

(1) **Get a blood test** to really know what is missing in your body and take action by feeding your body with the nutrients it lacks.

(2) **Positive Mindset**

Establish a positive **mindset** daily. I am sure you have heard or seen the following quote before:

"Whether you believe you can, or you believe you can't, you are right".

In other words what we believe strongly in our mind, it will happen. I don't know about you, but I choose to believe that I can do anything I set my mind to. That's why it is very important to establish a positive mindset.

- **(3) Drink at least 8 glasses of water per day** and slowly wean yourself off soft drinks, energy drinks, alcohol, etc. They are poison for your liver and will build sick blood cells.

PLEASE stay away from diet or 'no sugar' added soft drinks. They are PURE poison for your liver. The sweetener they use in those are synthetic and your liver does not recognize them.

- **(4) Increase energy** by feeding your body with healthy food such as veggies, legumes, fruits, whole-grains and herbs designed to increase energy. Switch to green tea instead of Coffee loaded with sugar.

- **(5) Exercise daily** – at least 30 minutes per day, 5-6 days per week and break a sweat.

- **(6) Think positive** in order to get positive results in weight-loss and life in general. Believe in yourself, believe you can do this! You also have to want this bad enough!

(7) Practice patience and perseverance daily – Good things come to those who wait and persevere. We tend to give up just before the miracle happens. I know because I have been there myself…

(8) Eat plenty of life-giving veggies. They build healthy blood cells which in turn promote long life and health. Consider using a super greens powder everyday in your protein shake.

(9) A pinch of sugar. Our blood cells need glucose for energy. Stay away from 'added sugar' (refined sugar, artificial sweeteners, cakes, chocolate, sweets. Only have as a treat in small amounts).

(10) Weigh yourself once a week. It makes you aware of your progress and choices you make daily. Adjust and correct as needed.

(11) Get enough sleep, at least 8 hours. Sleep boosts your metabolism and controls cravings. If you are sleep deprived, it will throw your body in chaos, especially your hormones. If hormones are imbalanced it affects your thyroid and weight-loss will be almost impossible.

(12)   **Boost your metabolism** to burn more fat. This can be done by drinking lots of water, exercising daily and simply combining all the natural weight-loss ingredients I mention here into one strong foundation to form daily life-long habits.

(13)   **Prayer and Faith in God**. This is optional but it has helped me out the most. Without God's beautiful promises and the hope that each promise gives me, I couldn't have done it alone. He gave and continues to give me strength daily.

It is always best to start with the basics first, make these ingredients your daily healthy life-style habits and add onto these ingredients a few more in-depth steps that I share with you in '**My 18 Year Weight-loss Journey**' book.

You will soon reach your weight-loss goal and live a much healthier, happier life as well as influence others around you to get healthy and fit.

The hardest obstacle I have found to get in the way is discouragement. It is because weight-loss is meant to be slow and steady to have lasting results.

If you lose weight too fast, then you will probably put it back on even faster because it simply is not healthy for the body to shed fat too fast. This is where you need patience and perseverance, which we have covered earlier.

Don't ever be tempted to give up, instead, enjoy the journey and everything that comes with it. When discouragement plagues your mind then start imagining 'healing' and the benefits that come with it.

It's also helpful to focus on the daily positive outcomes as a result of your newly adapted healthy lifestyle. Write down each positive you notice each day and then go over the list of positives whenever you are discouraged.

I always like to think of the turtle. She is slow but she keeps on moving constantly and gets to where she wants to go. She knows what she wants and where she wants to go and has patience.

Mindset is of the utmost importance and if you have it right then nothing will stop you.

There will come days of discouragement, temptations and negative thoughts, but armed with the right mindset and a strong foundation built of the ingredients I mentioned in this book, you will be ready and armed to face anything that comes your way.

With God, I have conquered huge mountains of anxiety, fear and depression. He invited me to give all my troubles, worries and fears to him and he promised me that if I do that, HE will give me rest.

It took years of pain, depression, fear and anxiety for me to learn to just trust him and leave it all in his hands. His beautiful promises definitely delivered.

Obesity is a tiresome heavy burden and can be a vicious cycle that holds you in a trap and you feel there is no way out. When I realized I can't do it on my own, I turned to God, my healer and he has definitely helped me out.

On the other hand, I had my important part to do which is feed my body with the foods that God intended for me, foods that will work with my body to heal it.

Junk food, soft drinks, alcohol and other harmful substances will only work against my body and bring disease and sickness on me.

I truly hope that this book has been helpful and encouraging to you and hope that it will help you on your journey to a new healthy and fit life.

I need your feedback!

Thank you so much for taking the time to read my book and if you have enjoyed it and have found it helpful, please leave me an honest feedback so that others can benefit from this book and my experience.

To leave feedback to this book just go to: www.amazon.com/author/irinadura and click on the book image and leave your feedback in the feedback section.

NOTE: Make sure you look for the book version that is currently available and in print. The version that is currently in print shows the price of the book. Ignore the earlier versions that are out of print and don't show a price.

Thank you so much for your precious time and God bless you with health, peace, happiness and long life!

Thank you

Before and After - From 100.1kg to 65Kg in 15 months.

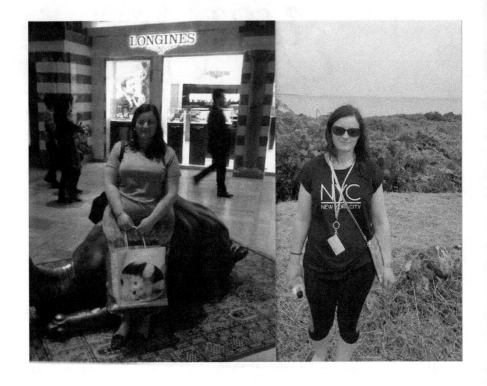

Me – Before and After.

notes

May 2014	May 2016
Waist: 113 cm	Waist: 81 cm
Hips: 130 cm	Hips: 95 cm
Bust: 115 cm	Bust: 98 cm
Thigh: 72 cm	Thigh: 62 cm

My before and after measurements

If you would like to know more about my weight-loss experience and struggle you can read all about it in "**My 18 Year Weight-loss Journey**" available in E- book or Paperback.

NOTE: For paperback, make sure you select the current edition that is showing a price for the book and is currently in print. Ignore the earlier versions that show 'Out of print – Limited availability'.

Go to: **www.amazon.com/author/irinadura** to purchase your copy. You will learn from my experience and mistakes and be motivated to start your healthy lifestyle journey.

If you know someone that would benefit from my books, please share my books with them or why not make it a special gift for the ones you care about ☐

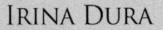

IRINA DURA

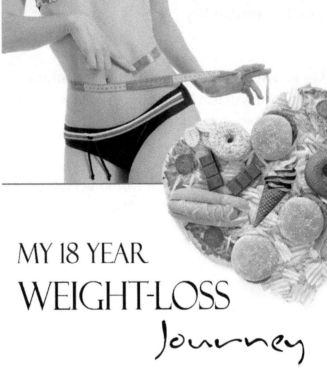

MY 18 YEAR
WEIGHT-LOSS
Journey

How I finally lost 35kg (77 pounds) while still enjoying my favorite food

In 'My Natural Weight-loss Recipe' the Author shares her basic list of ingredients that has laid down the sure foundation for her final weight-loss victory. The first ingredient on her list is 'Blood test' and for a very good reason. Feeling tired, heavy and in pain everyday prompted her to see her doctor who suggested a blood test. The results of that blood test opened her eyes to the danger she was in and how her bad habits were digging her an early grave. She was told she must do something about her weight or she will face Diabetes and other life-threatening diseases very soon.

She wasn't going to accept a life of sickness and disease and so she worked out a strategy to finally reach her weight-loss goal. Using her strategy she was able to lose 77 pounds within 15 months and wrote about her experience in 'My 18 Year Weight-loss Journey'.

Her passion is to help, motivate and inspire others that are struggling with obesity and hopes that through sharing her experience she will change many lives. In this book you will discover her basic ingredients to natural, safe weight-loss. Once each ingredient is implemented and followed daily it lays the foundation to long-term weight-loss and a lifetime of healthy habits.

My passion is to help others live a healthier, happier life. I believe that we can do anything if we really set our mind to it.

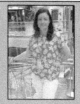

www.purenutritiondaily.com

Biography
Health
Motivational
Self improvement
Weight loss

www.ingramcontent.com/pod-product-compliance
Lightning Source LLC
LaVergne TN
LVHW021029171224
799328LV00009B/509